Cambridge Elements

Elements of Improving Quality and Safety in Healthcare
edited by
Mary Dixon-Woods,* Katrina Brown,* Sonja Marjanovic,†
Tom Ling,† Ellen Perry,* Graham Martin,* Gemma Petley,*
and Claire Dipple*
*THIS Institute (The Healthcare Improvement Studies Institute)
†RAND Europe

EDUCATION AND TRAINING AS IMPROVEMENT INTERVENTIONS

Lauren E. Benishek, Albert W. Wu, and
Michael A. Rosen
Johns Hopkins University

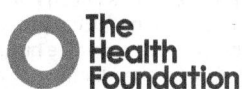

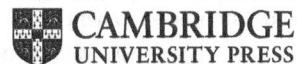

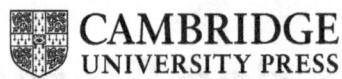

Shaftesbury Road, Cambridge CB2 8EA, United Kingdom

One Liberty Plaza, 20th Floor, New York, NY 10006, USA

477 Williamstown Road, Port Melbourne, VIC 3207, Australia

314–321, 3rd Floor, Plot 3, Splendor Forum, Jasola District Centre, New Delhi – 110025, India

103 Penang Road, #05–06/07, Visioncrest Commercial, Singapore 238467

Cambridge University Press is part of Cambridge University Press & Assessment, a department of the University of Cambridge.

We share the University's mission to contribute to society through the pursuit of education, learning and research at the highest international levels of excellence.

www.cambridge.org
Information on this title: www.cambridge.org/9781009326346

DOI: 10.1017/9781009326308

© THIS Institute 2025

This publication is in copyright. Subject to statutory exception and to the provisions of relevant collective licensing agreements, with the exception of the Creative Commons version the link for which is provided below, no reproduction of any part may take place without the written permission of Cambridge University Press & Assessment.

An online version of this work is published at doi.org/10.1017/9781009326308 under a Creative Commons Open Access license CC-BY-NC-ND 4.0 which permits re-use, distribution and reproduction in any medium for non-commercial purposes providing appropriate credit to the original work is given. You may not distribute derivative works without permission. To view a copy of this license, visit https://creativecommons.org/licenses/by-nc-nd/4.0

When citing this work, please include a reference to the DOI 10.1017/9781009326308

First published 2025

A catalogue record for this publication is available from the British Library

ISBN 978-1-009-32634-6 Paperback
ISSN 2754-2912 (online)
ISSN 2754-2904 (print)

Cambridge University Press & Assessment has no responsibility for the persistence or accuracy of URLs for external or third-party internet websites referred to in this publication and does not guarantee that any content on such websites is, or will remain, accurate or appropriate.

Every effort has been made in preparing this Element to provide accurate and up-to-date information which is in accord with accepted standards and practice at the time of publication. Although case histories are drawn from actual cases, every effort has been made to disguise the identities of the individuals involved. Nevertheless, the authors, editors and publishers can make no warranties that the information contained herein is totally free from error, not least because clinical standards are constantly changing through research and regulation. The authors, editors and publishers therefore disclaim all liability for direct or consequential damages resulting from the use of material contained in this Element. Readers are strongly advised to pay careful attention to information provided by the manufacturer of any drugs or equipment that they plan to use.

For EU product safety concerns, contact us at Calle de José Abascal, 56, 1°, 28003 Madrid, Spain, or email eugpsr@cambridge.org

Education and Training as Improvement Interventions

Elements of Improving Quality and Safety in Healthcare

DOI: 10.1017/9781009326308
First published online: December 2025

Lauren E. Benishek, Albert W. Wu, and Michael A. Rosen
Johns Hopkins University
Author for correspondence: Michael A. Rosen, mrosen44@jhmi.edu

Abstract: Delivering safe, high-quality care needs a competent and capable workforce, particularly as clinical practices change with scientific and technical advances. Structured learning opportunities are a central approach to building and maintaining competencies, but ineffective training wastes the scarce resources and staff time. This Element provides a review of education and training design, implementation, and evaluation methods used in healthcare improvement. Drawing from the general learning sciences and healthcare education and training literatures, the authors describe five pillars of effective training. For each pillar, they provide actionable guidance based on the best available evidence. Three examples of quality and safety programmes are given to illustrate the positive impact of well-designed training, and the challenges of good training design in healthcare improvement. This title is also available as open access on Cambridge Core.

Keywords: training design, training evaluation, competency, assessment, education and curriculum development

© THIS Institute 2025

ISBNs: 9781009326346 (PB), 9781009326308 (OC)
ISSNs: 2754-2912 (online), 2754-2904 (print)

Contents

1	Introduction	1
2	A Brief History of Training Research	1
3	How Can Education and Training Be Used to Support Healthcare Improvement?	5
4	Education and Training in Action	18
5	Critiques of Training as an Improvement Approach	23
6	Conclusions	25
7	Further Reading	26
	Contributors	27
	References	29

1 Introduction

For safe and high-quality healthcare, the people working in the system need diverse expertise – including but not limited to the fundamental technical skills required to implement a best practice and adapt as needed,[1] teamwork skills to coordinate care,[2] the attitudes and behaviours underlying a robust safety culture,[3] and the leadership skills to bring about change and improvement.[4] Education and training are therefore foundational approaches in healthcare improvement.

Education and training both describe the systematic provision of instruction intended to teach new competencies (knowledge, skills, and attitudes) to learners. Education generally refers to broader and more fundamental instruction taking place within degree-granting and continuing education programmes. Training refers to instruction with a narrower scope, targeting competencies within a specific task, technology, or improvement project. In this Element, our primary focus is on training as a component of interventions aimed at specific healthcare improvement efforts, though we do also consider broader education within the health professions.[5] Our emphasis is on evidence-based practices of training design, implementation, and evaluation.

In the following sections, we:

- identify historical and current trends in the science and practice of education and training for quality and safety
- detail evidence-based principles and practices for developing, implementing, and evaluating training interventions
- provide case examples of how education and training have been applied to healthcare improvement efforts
- critically examine the current state of research and practice, highlighting productive avenues for future research and innovation.

2 A Brief History of Training Research

Multidisciplinary improvement studies and professional education research literatures have generated a broad and deep knowledge base. A complete overview of this topic would fill many volumes on specific topics such as needs analysis, evaluation,[6] specific learning strategies,[7,8] and overall systems of training[9] and educational design[10], and is beyond the scope of this Element. Here, we review some key trends in this research and then briefly summarise developments in education and training for healthcare improvement.

2.1 Trends in Training Research

Researchers have studied training in organisations widely for over a century.[11] Early efforts were less than ideal: a landmark review characterised the state of the research up to 1970 as 'voluminous, nonempirical, nontheoretical, poorly written, and dull'.[12] Much has changed in the past 50 years, and there is now a rich theory-driven and empirical literature to inform the development, implementation, and evaluation of education and training programmes.[13–18] Practical implications of this work are discussed in detail in Section 3. Next, we highlight four key trends.

First, early research on training evaluation focused heavily on trainee reactions (e.g. self-reported learner perceptions of the training). This slowed down progress in the field; training reactions demonstrate negligible associations with outcomes of more value to organisations, such as behaviour change and improved performance[19] and are more related to learner characteristics (e.g. motivation to learn, anxiety) than to the training itself.[20] Over time, researchers have grown more sophisticated in how they view training effectiveness, with a focus on its multidimensional, multilevel, and dynamic nature (Box 1).

Second, it is now clear that education and training outcomes are influenced by a wide range of learner characteristics, including motivation, self-efficacy, goal orientation, age, cognitive ability, values and perceptions of organisational support and climate, among many others.[11,17] As a result, strategies to adapt training

---

Box 1 Attributes of training effectiveness to consider in evaluating training

Multidimensional: cognitive (e.g. knowledge, strategies), skill or behavioural (e.g. psychomotor or procedural skills), and affective (e.g. reactions to training, attitudinal changes) outcomes based on the objectives of a training programme. Often, training will target multiple dimensions concurrently.

Multilevel: impact of training individuals, teams, and larger organisational units is assessed. Assessing the impact on overall organisational performance remains a critical challenge for the field.[21]

Dynamic: outcomes may change at different rates and therefore should be looked at over different timescales. For example, evaluation of team training interventions in healthcare indicates faster improvements for cognitive and behavioural outcomes, but slower changes for attitudinal outcomes (e.g. it takes longer for learners to adjust their beliefs in the importance of teamwork or team cohesion).[22]

design for the unique characteristics of learners or to allow for increased learner control over their experiences have been developed. Self-directed learning, where learners take an active role in planning and executing their own training, is at least as effective as more traditional methods.[23] However, the focus on learner characteristics has also resulted in notable missteps. Specifically, the strategy of accommodating different learner styles (e.g. preferences for learning modalities – the way in which individuals receive, give, and store information), while often deployed, lacks empirical support. People do consistently express preferences for different learning modalities, but aligning learning modalities with different preferences does not result in better learning outcomes.[24,25]

Third, the importance of context is increasingly well recognised: education and training do not occur in a vacuum. Factors within organisations – such as peer and leader support, culture, and opportunities to apply what was learned – impact on training effectiveness,[17, 26] for example, by affecting learners' pre-training and post-training motivation.[17] What happens in the learning environment (e.g. classroom, simulation centre, and online learning platform) is important, but what happens to learners before and after a training session matters just as much, and a comprehensive approach to managing training effectiveness needs to account for this. This has led training researchers to call for systems-based approaches to managing training design and delivery.

Fourth, decades of empirical work and theory development have yielded a broad evidence base to guide training design. Multiple versions of integrated instructional principles and methods now exist,[15–17,27] but they share many commonalities as they translate the same evidence base into practical approaches to training design. One such practically focused synthesis of the training literature is presented in Section 3, where we describe five pillars of effective training.

2.2 Recent Trends in Training to Improve the Quality and Safety of Healthcare

The increased emphasis on healthcare quality and safety in policy, practice, and research over the past couple of decades has been accompanied by reform and modernisation initiatives in health profession education. At the same time, a wide variety of training programmes have emerged seeking to target quality and safety-related competencies, both broad, such as communication and safety culture, and narrow, such as protocols for reducing risks of specific preventable harms.

One important move involves incorporation of quality and safety-related competencies into overall professional competency models and professional development.[28] Competency models are specifications of knowledge, skills, abilities, and other characteristics required for effective performance in a specific job, role, or task.[29] Training can be, for example, on systems-based care, evidence-based practice, or interprofessional communication and teamwork.[30,31] Overall, increased formalisation of safety and quality-related competencies is a positive development. However, initial efforts to define quality and safety-related competencies occurred within particular disciplines or geographical areas, resulting in inconsistent content and terminology.[30,32] More recent efforts have focused on developing international and interprofessional competencies for general areas like evidence-based practice,[33] as well as competencies related to specific types or sources of preventable harm, such as diagnostic error.[34] The quality and integration of these competency models are improving, with many resources to support them available. The process of developing and integrating competency models is still not complete and is likely to continue to mature while major questions – for example, about the extent to which there should be standards for all or a mix of standardised and unique competencies capturing the diverse work of different professionals – are addressed.

Another trend seen is in the growth of healthcare improvement projects intended to integrate quality and safety competencies into undergraduate and graduate health professional education.[35,36] When disconnected from clinical care delivery, these projects may limit both the learning opportunities and organisational benefit.[37] Recent approaches seek to more tightly couple educational improvement projects and organisational priorities. This is achieved through broader stakeholder engagement and participation, including both health system leaders[38] and patients[39] and through tighter linkage between formalised quality and safety curricula and practice-based learning experiences within organisations.[40] The gap between educational programmes and clinical care delivery systems has not been closed, but there is progress.

Recent years have also seen the expansion of the modes through which training is delivered and made accessible. Quality and safety training can take many forms, including those that are information-based (such as traditional lectures), demonstration-based (such as video-based examples, role-modelling), or practice-based (such as simulation-based training) methods.[41] The rise of simulation-based training has been a notable feature of recent years (see the Element on simulation as an improvement technique[42]). Immersive and interactive experiential learning is a powerful approach, but is resource-intensive, requiring significant investments in infrastructure, such as physical space, costly simulators, and faculty development. Many professionals lack the opportunity to participate in high-fidelity simulations, so scalable and cost-effective methods of simulation-based training for both high-resource and low-resource settings are an active area of development. For example, team training programmes often employ in-person simulation-based training, but one possible way of increasing scalability is to replace practice with demonstration (i.e. videos of simulations) and debriefing.[43] Other strategies to improve accessibility of learning opportunities include embedded and real-time or 'just-in-time' training (extremely brief reviews of content provided as needed in the work environment[44,45]). The COVID-19 pandemic posed several challenges to traditional education and training delivery approaches – limitations on in-person gatherings, a rapid pace of change as best practice evolved – and consequently accelerated the adoption of these 'just in time' learning approaches.[46,47]

A further major trend has been the recognition of the role of organisations in preparing their managers and leaders for the specialised expertise needed to support healthcare improvement.[48] Hospitals and health systems have increasingly become more active in this regard, for example, by formalising competencies across roles and areas of the organisation and ensuring everyone has the skills they need to fulfil their role. Management skills for healthcare improvement involve fluency with a wide range of process modelling and analysis tools, improvement cycles, financial planning, and programme evaluation methods, among others.[49,50]

Leadership for healthcare improvement requires a specific skillset that includes the ability to engage with others intellectually and emotionally, create a shared vision, negotiation, and conflict management. Important here is the distinction between 'hard' and 'soft' skills[51] in healthcare improvement education and training, which is consistent with many long-standing distinctions in the organisational sciences such as Heifetz's technical work (problems with relatively clear solutions that can be arrived at with existing knowledge of experts) and adaptive work (problems requiring developing novel solutions),[52] or Kotter's definitions of management (an organisation's approach to complexity) and leadership (an organisation's approach to change).[53] For both management and leadership, there is nothing easy about 'soft' skills[54]: they are often among the most challenging competencies to master.

3 How Can Education and Training Be Used to Support Healthcare Improvement?

In this section, we describe the core elements of training design and the application to healthcare improvement. Training is more than a singular event (or series of events, such as a workshop or semester/term-long course): it is a process beginning before a learning event takes place and continuing beyond the event's conclusion. Much needs to happen before, during, and after the learning event to maximise a training programme's usefulness, applicability, and effectiveness. Salas and colleagues[27] extracted five unifying themes from thousands of published best practices. Taken together, these themes – labelled 'pillars' – capture fundamental activities that are supported by evidence, as follows:

(1) ensure training is appropriate
(2) create a positive learning environment
(3) design and implement training to be accessible, useable, and effective
(4) evaluate training
(5) transfer and sustain competencies.

These themes are drawn from the broad interdisciplinary literature of the learning sciences; they are not specific to healthcare safety and quality applications but are rooted in theories and principles of human learning. While the safety and quality improvement field grows in the sophistication of its application of this science, recent reviews of training as applied to specific clinical tasks often indicate the existing literature is of low quality, and challenging to synthesise into actionable guidance.[55,56] Figure 1 depicts the five pillars spanning the before, during, and after stages of training, with important activities under each pillar presented as principles for action in Table 1. These evidence-based principles describe what should happen, and why, throughout the training process. Though we present them in sequential order, the activities within the pillars are, in reality, often iterative and interconnected. For example, results from training evaluation – Pillar 4 – might feed back into understanding training needs – Pillar 1.

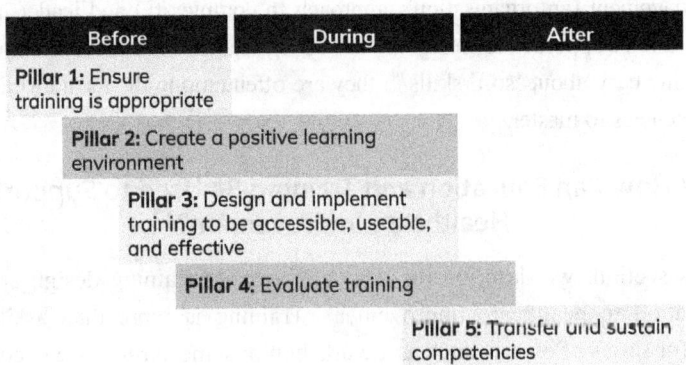

Figure 1 An overview of the pillars of training
Adapted from Gregory et al.[57]

Table 1 Evidence-based principles for successful healthcare improvement interventions

Pillar 1: Ensure training is appropriate	
Principle 1	Conduct a systematic training needs analysis
Principle 2	Confirm that training is an appropriate solution
Pillar 2: Create a positive learning environment	
Principle 3	Generate support from organisational leadership
Principle 4	Prepare participants for training
Principle 5	Respect participants' time and expertise
Pillar 3: Design and implement training to be accessible, useable, and effective	
Principle 6	Design training using evidence-based practices
Principle 7	Employ pedagogically sound instructional strategies
Pillar 4: Evaluate training	
Principle 8	Decide what to measure
Principle 9	Determine how to measure
Principle 10	Analyse evaluation data to assess training success
Pillar 5: Transfer and sustain competencies	
Principle 11	Facilitate the use of competencies in the work environment
Principle 12	Foster continual improvement and use of competencies
Principle 13	Improve training

3.1 Pillar 1: Ensure Training Is Appropriate

Training is a powerful tool in the healthcare improvement toolbox, but it is certainly not the only one. The first pillar is therefore to ensure that training is an appropriate intervention. This involves Principle 1 (conduct a systematic training needs analysis) and Principle 2 (confirm that training is an appropriate solution, or component of a broader solution).

3.1.1 Principle 1: Conduct a Systematic Training Needs Analysis

A needs analysis is the process of collecting relevant information about the organisation, department, or unit experiencing a safety or quality concern, the people involved in the issue, and the tasks related to the problem.[58–60] It informs decisions about what to train, how to train, who to train, and what factors might affect training success. A training needs analysis might build on the results of a root cause analysis by informing the content, scope, and application of a training programme. A needs analysis comprises three main components (see Box 2).[61,62]

> **BOX 2 THREE PRIMARY COMPONENTS OF A NEEDS ANALYSIS**
>
> **Task analysis** answers the question: What needs to be trained for? It determines job elements, details task requirements, and identifies the specific competencies (knowledge, skills, and attitudes – KSAs) required to successfully complete a job or task.
>
> **Person analysis** answers the questions: Who needs to be trained and what are their characteristics? It assesses who has (and who lacks) the competencies needed to perform a task successfully, and it may be used to identify who would most benefit from training and what training approaches might be best for the audience.
>
> **Organisational analysis** assesses strategic alignment with training and environmental readiness by answering the questions: What are the organisation's priorities? Is it ready for training? What possible barriers to successful training exist? It is an investigation into the strategies, culture, norms, limitations, resources, and stakeholder (e.g. leadership, frontline staff, and patients) support of training. An organisational analysis does not have to be a system-wide investigation; it may be limited to understanding the dynamics in a specific unit or department within a hospital or practice system.

3.1.2 Principle 2: Confirm That Training Is an Appropriate Solution

Deciding whether training is appropriate as a primary or supplementary intervention to support improvement is critical. Though not validated across healthcare broadly, hierarchies of control or intervention effectiveness have been developed across industries[63] and for different types of risks in healthcare including infection prevention[64] and medication safety.[65] For example, the USA's National Institute for Occupational Safety and Health (NIOSH)'s hierarchy of controls identifies five types of control that can be used to avoid exposures to safety hazards.[64] These controls, in decreasing order of effectiveness, include:

- elimination (physically removing the hazard)
- substitution (replacing the hazard)
- engineering (isolating people from the hazard)
- administrative (changing the way people work)
- personal protective equipment (PPE; providing barriers when encountering the hazard).

Administrative and PPE controls are often used when existing processes do not control hazards particularly well. As such, they are not as effective as other healthcare improvement strategies that require less effort from affected workers. Although training might be used to support or reinforce new procedures related to other types of control (e.g. PPE donning and doffing), training itself falls under the category of administrative control, and is considered a weaker form of intervention. Therefore, healthcare improvement practitioners should critically consider what additional interventions they may pair with training to comprehensively address safety issues. A further consideration is the often resource-intensive nature of training. It can be time-consuming, expensive, and logistically challenging to design, implement, and sustain, and single trainings are often insufficient for long-term change.[66] Therefore, when deciding whether training is appropriate, practitioners need to assess whether resources are available to do it well or whether other options might adequately address the problem.

The validity of the hierarchy of controls concept and its application to healthcare safety and quality is not universally accepted,[67] and should not be relied on in a rigid manner. However, the core idea is that improving quality and safety requires changing behaviour, that multiple types of interventions can facilitate that behaviour change, and that context will determine which methods, or combination thereof, will be most effective. For example, the long history of improving hand hygiene compliance demonstrates that, while knowledge of and skill performing hand sanitation is important, it is only part of a larger change solution involving foundational system changes (such as changing from soap to alcohol-based agents to reduce the time burden, physically locating sanitising stations to integrate with workflow).[68] These system changes need to be in place before training and other behaviour change interventions can have maximum effect. In practice, determining if, or to what degree, training should be a part of the change effort can be challenging. Task analysis methods[69], participatory design methods[70], and help to identify changes to task workflows, technology, physical spaces, or other work system redesigns may be beneficial.

3.2 Pillar 2: Create a Positive Learning Environment

Creating an environment conducive to learning can help in capitalising on training investment. A positive learning environment can be created in several ways, but important principles include generating support from organisational leadership, preparing participants for training, and respecting participants' time and expertise.

3.2.1 Principle 3: Generate Support from Organisational Leadership

Leadership support for training can take the form of investing financial and non-financial resources into the development, implementation, and sustainment of training initiatives as well as communicating the organisational value of training to learners. Learners' perceptions of leadership support for a training programme influence their perceptions of that programme's usefulness and transfer of training.[71,72] Consequently, early involvement of leaders in planning and designing a training intervention is critical. For example, the Comprehensive Unit-based Safety Program (CUSP) is a method for creating safer, higher-quality care through the combination of teamwork, clinical best practice, and safety science.[73,74] The CUSP team is interprofessional, consisting of nurses, physicians, facility or unit management, chief quality officers, and patient safety officers, among others. One key to CUSP's success has been the partnership between frontline providers and senior executives.

3.2.2 Principle 4: Prepare Participants for Training

Training effectiveness is improved when learners understand its purpose, objective, and expected outcomes.[75] Participants develop expectations before training, and those with unmet expectations demonstrate lower self-efficacy, motivation, and commitment to using trained competencies on the job.[76] Therefore, preparing participants requires communication early and often with them about the training purpose, who is required or invited to participate, why they have been invited, what they will experience, and when and how they will complete training.[14] All formal and informal communications should be clear, concise, and frame training positively. For example, training should be presented as an opportunity for growth rather than as punishment for mistakes or errors, and it should be discussed with enthusiasm rather than as an inconvenience. Participants should be encouraged to set quality and safety goals for themselves and their units to engage them prior to training.

3.2.3 Principle 5: Respect Participants' Time and Expertise

It is important for trainees to:[17,77]

- understand why they need to learn new competencies
- see the relevance of training and how these new competencies will help *them*, specifically (and not just the organisation)
- experience some level of internal motivation
- build on their prior knowledge and experiences during training
- have some autonomy with directing their own learning.

Education and Training as Improvement Interventions

In addition to Principle 4, it is helpful to establish ground rules in advance of training, particularly if the intervention is in person or takes place with others. Ground rules include framing practice errors positively (as an opportunity to learn what not to do) and suspending judgments of others. Such expectations can facilitate participant self-efficacy, or the belief that they are capable of meeting performance targets.[78]

3.3 Pillar 3: Design and Implement Training to Be Accessible, Usable, and Effective

Well-designed training should not present significant barriers or difficulty to participation (*accessibility*). It should be easy for participants to navigate and straightforward for instructors or facilitators to implement (*usability*) and promote maximum increases in targeted competencies (*effectiveness*).

3.3.1 Principle 6: Design Training Using Evidence-Based Practices

Subject matter expertise needed to inform the training content needs to be complemented by instructional design expertise in supporting the design process, including formulating learning objectives, establishing performance criteria, providing controlled learning experiences, conducting performance assessments, and providing helpful feedback.[16] Goldstein and Ford[16] provides an expansive overview of the training design and development process. Those using education and training as an improvement strategy should form partnerships with learning or instructional design professionals when integrating training into quality and safety initiatives.

Regardless of who is part of the instructional design team, the most fundamental step is to identify and describe the training goals as well-written learning objectives. Learning objectives state what learners are expected to be able to know, do, or feel upon completion of training.[10] Learning objectives should be drawn from needs analysis findings (Principle 1), which will inform the content scope (what needs to be trained) for the selected training audience (who needs to be trained). Desired training outcomes may focus on cognitive (knowledge-based), affective (emotion-based), or psychomotor (action/skill-based) changes and learning objectives can range in complexity. For example, cognitive learning may involve rote knowledge recall, comprehending new facts, applying facts to novel situations, analysing information into component parts, evaluating information and ideas for validity and quality, or synthesising information to build new understanding.[79,80] For these reasons, it can be difficult to write clear learning objectives. Many resources exist that offer guidance for crafting concrete and measurable objectives.[81]

Once finalised, learning objectives identify the specific competencies to be addressed in the training programme. Competencies are the required knowledge, skills, and attitudes (KSAs) an individual must possess to complete a particular task. Many examples of these competency models exist for healthcare quality and safety.

The Health Professions Education: A Bridge to Quality report[82] was produced in response to the Institute of Medicine's 2001 call for an interdisciplinary summit to outline reforms for health professional education to meet the challenges outlined in the Crossing the Quality Chasm Report.[83] The panel advocated that all health professional education programmes should prepare individuals to:

- provide patient-centred care
- work in interdisciplinary teams
- employ evidence-based practice
- apply quality improvement
- use informatics.

In 2006, the Canadian Patient Safety Institute (CPSI) designed The Safety Competencies for healthcare professionals.[7,34,37] The revised framework incorporates six patient safety domains:

- patient safety culture
- teamwork
- communication
- safety, risk, and quality improvement
- optimise human and system factors
- recognise, respond to, and disclose patient safety incidents.[84]

Under this framework, CPSI has identified numerous key and enabling competencies related to each of these six patient safety domains. The enabling competency statements describe concrete, measurable, and specific KSAs relevant to each of the patient safety domains which can be mapped to training programme learning objectives to facilitate a robust, evidence-based curriculum.

3.3.2 Principle 7: Employ Pedagogically Sound Instructional Strategies

Instructional strategies refer to the tools, methods, and context used in forming an overall approach to training delivery. A thorough training strategy incorporates four methods to guide, teach, and prepare learners, with each method strategically building on the other:

- information
- demonstration
- practice
- feedback.[13,14]

Training should provide the necessary *information* that learners need to be able to perform at a minimally acceptable level of competency. Precisely what and how much information is needed will be driven by needs analysis findings, but should always be made meaningful to learners. In the case of adult learners, it is critical, for example, that information is job-relevant and builds on their current expertise and experience – otherwise, training may lose their attention or waste their time. Beyond information, *demonstration* allows learners to observe behaviours, their results, and contextual cues. Social learning theory suggests that new behaviours can be learned by observing and imitating others.[85] Positive demonstrations showcase proficiency with a competency, while negative demonstrations show what does not work well. Both types allow learners to analyse behaviour and emulate what works and avoid what does not. Moreover, demonstration-based learning can be interactive, allowing training participants to discuss and analyse together the successes and failures of the models they observe.

Observation and information alone are unlikely to be sufficient strategies for helping learners reach proficiency with a competency: most KSAs require some amount of *practice* to master. Opportunities to enable learners to experiment with different behaviours and refine their own performance are therefore important. Practice in low-stakes environments where errors have minimal consequences are ideal situations for learners still new to a competency. Learners with more proficiency may benefit from higher-stakes practice situations in which they can be challenged to improve their performance under different stressors. Key to successful practice opportunities, no matter how novice the learner, is ensuring that the learning environment is physically and psychologically safe.[75]

Finally, constructive *feedback* – reinforcing, or corrective – is a critical complement to practice.[75] Reinforcing feedback confirms for the learner the desirability of their performance. Corrective feedback explains what was flawed about a learner's performance and offers suggestions for improvement. Some forms of training actively encourage mistakes to test competency progression and enhance learning. Error management training (EMT), for example, is a highly effective method that encourages trainees to explore their performance and make errors.[86–88] Errors are considered an expected consequence of active learning and can help instructors and learners identify competency gaps. An expected practical outcome of EMT is that trainees will learn how to manage errors in the moment.

In summary, practising newly learned KSAs in a physically and psychologically safe environment where learners can observe and interact with each other while receiving feedback from content experts, instructors, and peers helps to maximise learning.[75]

3.4 Pillar 4: Evaluate Training

Evaluation, the systematic collection of data to assess training effectiveness, informs understanding of whether quality and safety competencies have improved and how far change can be attributed to the training programme. Evaluation can refer to the effectiveness of the programme itself, where a training programme's strengths, weaknesses and usefulness for meeting organisational objectives are assessed. Evaluation can also refer to the learners, where assessing growth in participants' competencies allows for more targeted feedback or remediation tailored to participants' unique needs. These aims are important to articulate at the outset of evaluation planning, as they will drive choices of what and how to measure. The evaluation strategy should be developed and implemented alongside the training itself. Evaluation metrics should match learning objectives and capture specific KSAs. We offer three additional principles to guide evaluation strategies: Principle 8: Decide what to measure, Principle 9: Decide how to measure, and Principle 10: Analyse evaluation data to infer training success.

3.4.1 Principle 8: Decide What to Measure

Evaluation frameworks guide evaluation planning. Although many have been described, Kirkpatrick's[89,90] is among the most commonly used. It comprises four evaluation criteria domains:

- reactions
- learning
- transfer
- results.

Reactions refer to learners' attitudes towards the training programme, such as enjoyment (i.e. training satisfaction) and perceived usefulness (i.e. beliefs that they gained important new KSAs). *Learning* refers to changes in targeted competencies because of training participation. Often, learning assessment is where many training evaluations begin and end, but the next level of evaluation criteria, *transfer*, will be critically important for patient safety improvement initiatives. *Transfer* (also known as *behaviours*) describes learners' application of new patient safety competencies to their work environment. *Results* refer to the organisational benefit achieved because of training. Results expected from patient safety training initiatives might include improved workflow, reduced

Education and Training as Improvement Interventions

burnout, shorter hospital length of stay, or any other number of desirable outcomes. Typically, results only manifest when acquired competencies are transferred to the work environment. Results can include patient outcomes, though including measures more proximal to the behaviour change in addition to patient outcomes is advisable. Phillips extended Kirkpatrick's model by including a 'return on investment' (ROI) domain,[91–93] a measure of how much the organisation saves on costs as a result of training. The ROI is frequently driven by results (e.g. fewer medical errors or malpractice lawsuits).

These training outcomes can be measured in several ways. Good, content-relevant measures will inform performance diagnosis (i.e. understanding the reasons why behaviour may or may not have changed) and meaningful and constructive feedback. Measurement can be useful before and during (not only after) training, particularly during practice opportunities. Measures that target the specific competencies framed in the objectives will offer the most precise estimate of the training's usefulness. Similarly, organisational results should be linked to training learning objectives. For example, if training was intended to help providers navigate an electronic health record more efficiently, it may be reasonable to expect a decrease in burnout in the long term. However, it may be less appropriate to expect a reduction in surgical site infections.

3.4.2 Principle 9: Decide How to Measure

When thinking about *what* to measure, it is easy to begin to consider *how* it will be measured. As with the other principles, choosing how to measure should be tied to what, precisely, it is that training is intended to improve. Section 2.1 introduced training evaluation outcomes. Some types of learning outcomes lend themselves naturally to certain measurement methods. For example, data on training reactions (i.e. learners' perceptions of the quality and value of the learning experience, and their ability to apply what they've learned) may be suited to self-reported responses to Likert-style rating scales (i.e. standard surveys). Learning – the knowledge, skills, and attitudes changed by the learning experience – may be captured using some form of declarative knowledge or situation judgement test (i.e. specialised surveys asking people how they would respond in different situations).[94] Learning and transfer can be measured observationally, either during simulation exercises or on the job through trained observers, supervisors, or peer assessments.

Measures that capture both outcomes and processes are also important. Changes in processes often precede changes in outcomes, so measuring both will give a finer understanding of where quality and safety competencies are being enacted. In a systematic review of the literature, Okuyama and colleagues identified 34 published tools for assessing patient safety competencies, including teamwork, risk management, and communication.[95] Choosing validated measures aligned to targeted KSAs (Principle 6) from among this toolkit of existing metrics is a good starting point for developing a training programme evaluation plan.

3.4.3 Principle 10: Analyse Evaluation Data to Assess Training Success

After collecting various types of evaluation criteria (e.g. reactions, learning, transfer, and results, see Principle 9), data can be used to understand whether training has been successful and why. The descriptive and analytical methods appropriate for assessing training success will depend on the types of data collected and the goals of analysis. For more details on precisely how to use statistical methods to analyse training evaluation data, see references such as Philips and Philips.[92] The interpretation of the findings will guide the next steps (e.g. sustaining new competencies, strengthening the training programme).

3.5 Pillar 5: Transfer and Sustain Competencies

While structured training events have a distinct start and end point, the learning process is ongoing, involving competency transfer to new environments, repetition to strengthen newly formed skills and attitudes, and continued use or refreshers to sustain performance. The following three principles support transfer and sustainability.

3.5.1 Principle 11: Facilitate the Use of Competencies in the Work Environment

Learning without transfer to the work environment does not secure improvement, but transfer is not an automatic extension of learning. Special effort must be made to promote the application and adoption of new competencies at work.[71] Encouraging the application of trained KSAs requires organisational support – even a single disparaging comment about training (e.g. 'That was a waste of your time') can halt transfer.[96] Therefore, healthcare improvement practitioners, organisational leadership, and unit management need to be highly intentional in encouraging, reinforcing, and even modelling the desired behaviours. Such behaviours send strong signals about what is expected in the organisation, increasing the likelihood that similar behaviours will be adopted by other employees.[97]

A lack of opportunities to use new skills is one of the strongest barriers to transfer.[98] Learners need to be given plenty of opportunities to use their new KSAs, as otherwise skill decay may occur.[99] Feedback remains important in transferring KSAs, as well as creating comfort and dexterity with them. Even though these opportunities may be real-life events and not simply 'practice' opportunities, learners need to be encouraged to voice questions or comments regarding the appropriate use of KSAs. Practice should be as soon as possible after training events. Where it is not possible to practice immediately, for example, if training is intended to address competencies needed during rare events, dialogue may be important to preventing decay.

3.5.2 Principle 12: Foster Continuous Improvement and Use of Competencies

Training may, in principle, create long-term or permanent changes in competencies. But sustaining newly acquired KSAs requires consistent use, reinforcement, and correction to mitigate skill decay.[100] The beneficial impact of training can be sustained for a longer duration with regular attention to performance through strategies like team debriefings and reward systems.[17] Debriefings are meetings during which employees can evaluate their performance as a team, offering suggestions for improvement and recognising successful use of KSAs.[101] Recognition can be a powerful driver for perpetuating desired behaviour.[102] Showcasing 'bright spots' (teams or individuals who have done an exceptional job demonstrating valued competencies) can reinforce behaviour among both individuals being recognised and other organisational members. Finally, embedding quality and safety competencies as part of the organisational reward structure can also help promote long-term sustainment of competencies. Recognising and promoting individuals based on safe practice helps to formalise performance expectations.

3.5.3 Principle 13: Improve Training

Data collected from training evaluation may point to weak spots within the training curriculum itself. Perhaps the programme was not well-suited to the audience (either because the learning objectives were too simple or too advanced) or minimal shifts in learning, transfer, or results were seen. It will be critical to assess whether failures to see desired outcomes are due to the training curriculum or some other explanation (e.g. an incompatible organisational culture). Updating training format, methods, and content in response to evaluation findings may be an ongoing, but necessary, process. Otherwise, using inadequate or outdated training curricula becomes a waste of organisational resources. While often an informal learning process, several formal approaches for training redesign and continuous improvement have been proposed. These include methods that incorporate content experts' ratings of the importance of competencies included in training, and cyclically re-establishing training needs to ensure existing training is addressing those needs.[103]

4 Education and Training in Action

The principles detailed previously outline a rigorous and evidence-based approach to training design. In this section, we describe two cases where education and training played a critical role in a healthcare improvement initiative, illustrating both the importance of education and training and the common challenges faced. They show how, like any design process, training design is often iterative, adapted to manage constraints, and deviates from the idealised process. The first example of the Practical Obstetric Multi-Professional Training (PROMPT) programme describes a pure training intervention (i.e. the main intervention is skill building) which has been widely adopted and evaluated. The second two cases are from the authors' experience and demonstrate how training is integrated as a part of multicomponent quality and safety improvement interventions.

4.1 Improving Obstetric Emergency Outcomes for Mothers and Babies

The Practical Obstetric Multi-Professional Training programme is an internationally implemented training programme designed to build the individual and team skills needed to effectively respond to obstetric emergencies.[104] The programme began in 2006 at Southmead Hospital in Bristol, United Kingdom. The course directors of an obstetrics emergency training day conducted a post hoc evaluation of the programme's impact on maternal and neonatal outcomes, finding substantial improvement across measures in the post-implementation period.[105] This programme was further refined and evaluated in the Simulation and Fire-drill Evaluation randomised controlled trial, which demonstrated a positive impact on both team and technical performance.[106] From there, the PROMPT training was packaged for broader regional, national, and international dissemination.

The appropriateness of training as a solution, and specific competencies targeted (Pillar 1), were initially established through observed gaps in adherence to best practice responses to infrequent but critical obstetric emergencies. Childbirth is a heavily litigated area, and evidence from cases where best practice was not followed has informed the development of PROMPT and similar training programmes.[107] PROMPT focuses on two distinct sets of competencies: evidence-based interventions for the management of obstetric emergencies, and team skills needed to manage these stressful environments

Education and Training as Improvement Interventions   19

and time-critical tasks. The technical competencies include the knowledge and skills required to perform evidence-based best practice care for an annually updated list of conditions such as shoulder dystocia (where one or both shoulders get stuck during labour), neonatal resuscitation, vaginal breach births, maternal sepsis, and cord prolapse. The teamwork skills drew from general principles of crew resource management first introduced in aviation and subsequently adapted and broadly adopted in healthcare.[108]

PROMPT employs methods that are both information-based (a comprehensive training guide including information on the evidence behind emergency management) and simulation-based, giving learners the opportunity to practice technical and teamwork skills in a controlled environment, and participate in team debriefs to facilitate learning (Pillar 3).[109] PROMPT has undergone numerous rigorous evaluations (Pillar 4), and has demonstrated impact on teamwork climate, neonatal outcomes, and maternal outcomes.[110] Somewhat uniquely for training programmes targeting quality and safety, it has also shown financial return on investment (reduction in litigation expenses).[107] Finally, the recommended training model for PROMPT requires annual retraining of 100 per cent of ward staff, emphasising the need to sustain training gains with recurring opportunities to refresh previously learned skills and understand changes to evidence-based management strategies as the underlying literature evolves (Pillar 5). Managing this sustainment over time requires organisational support across many levels of leadership.[111]

The success of PROMPT is impressive and encouraging for the value of training as a solution to important quality and safety challenges. A systematic review and meta-analysis of the broader obstetric emergency team training literature indicated mixed evidence and suggested that programmes employing in situ team simulations demonstrated the most benefit.[112] This underscores the importance of choosing appropriate methods of training delivery (Pillar 3).

4.2 Improving Paediatric Cardiopulmonary Resuscitation

Approximately 6,000 children have an in-hospital cardiac arrest every year in the United States. While there have been marked improvements in outcomes in recent years, most children do not survive. However, there are large differences in survival between facilities, indicating potential for improvement. In 2013, the Johns Hopkins Hospital set a goal of improving adherence to the American Heart Association's Paediatric Advanced Life Support chest compression guidelines. Full details of the programme to achieve this goal are available elsewhere,[113] but in the following, we describe the overall programme structure and the critical role training played in achieving consistent increase in the quality of cardiopulmonary resuscitation (CPR) for children.

The healthcare improvement programme began by developing key infrastructure for a learning process. A data surveillance system was created to identify any potential in-hospital cardiac arrests through code button pushes, rapid response team activations, electronic health records, and billing codes for CPR. Subsequently, a data capture system to investigate each potential event and centralise all performance data for events verified to be in-hospital cardiac arrests was created. This infrastructure was key to defining performance gaps, and as a source of evaluation data (Pillar 4). A weekly debriefing meeting was established to discuss all verified cardiac arrest resuscitations from the preceding week, based on the principle that debriefing is an effective method of learning from collective experience.[101,114] The effectiveness of debriefing relies on establishing a psychological safe learning environment for people to question assumptions and voice their perspectives, which was achieved in these meetings through introductions to the session and debrief facilitation practices aimed at promoting trust and openness (Pillar 2).[115]

The data-informed debriefing process was extremely effective at surfacing challenges and generating potential solutions. Over time, these issues and ideas were organised into themes, evaluated for efficacy, and integrated into the ongoing cycle of training and certification for Paediatric Advanced Life Support and other reinforcing training activities (e.g. in situ simulations) if proven effective. Specifically, action-linked phrases, choreography, and ergonomics were three components of the resuscitation quality improvement bundle developed from debrief lessons learned.

First, action-linked phrases combined call-outs (e.g. 'there's no pulse') and task delegation (e.g. 'start compressions'), two widely recognised patterns of high-functioning teams. This addressed the common pattern observed in resuscitation events where team members would share critical information, but others would fail to respond to it. The effectiveness of training using action-linked phrases was demonstrated in simulation.[116] Second, choreography involved defining structured plans for how the resuscitation team should interact physically with one another, the room, and their equipment. Variations of choreography were explored in simulations, and a gold standard was established.[117] A video of this gold standard was created and used in future training sessions. Third, ergonomics of room layouts and equipment were thoroughly assessed, and modifications made where appropriate and practical (e.g. redesign of resuscitation carts).

Action-linked phrases and choreography relied mostly on behavioural competencies of the team members, so training was chosen as a primary intervention in addition to cognitive aids (i.e. graphic and textual depictions of resuscitation algorithms). Training, which included practice opportunities for action-linked phrases, choreography, and ergonomics during simulated resuscitation events, extended learning beyond the group participating in the debrief, as important innovations were codified into new curricula and integrated into existing training opportunities. This served to spread lessons learned as far as possible, but also to minimise the training burden on staff (e.g. a new training programme wasn't developed, but new learning objectives and competencies were integrated into existing learning opportunities; Pillar 5).

4.3 The Resilience in Stressful Events (RISE) Programme

Health workers involved in adverse events, including medical errors, often experience serious harm themselves. The term 'second victim' was first coined in 2000 to describe healthcare providers who are involved in an incident in which a patient is harmed, and who may be emotionally traumatised as a result.[118] Common emotional responses include grief, anxiety, guilt, fear, and loss of confidence. Workers may experience flashbacks and disturbed sleep, and symptoms can sometimes progress to post-traumatic stress disorder (PTSD). In the short term, the functioning of affected workers may be impaired, and some may develop burnout. Health workers can also be traumatised by other stressful events, such as a patient's death, unexpected complication, conflict with family members, or workplace violence.[119] Studies have found that up to half of workers have experienced the second victim syndrome, and the majority are not supported by their institutions.

To address this gap, in 2011, the Johns Hopkins Hospital instituted the Resilience in Stressful Events (RISE) peer support programme.[120] After a stressful patient-related event, health workers can call RISE using the hospital's intranet or electronic paging system, 24 hours a day, 7 days a week. Peer responders are volunteers who work in the hospital and include a diverse group of nurses, physicians, social workers, chaplains, pharmacists, technicians, first responders, and others. The on-call peer-responder calls back immediately and schedules a meeting. Meetings are often scheduled at the end of a shift, can be in-person or virtual, and can accommodate an individual or a group.[121] Responders provide psychological first aid and emotional support. The responder also provides information on organisational resources, such as the internal employee assistance programme, or external resources like community counsellors. Encounters are completely confidential, and reports are not shared with managers, risk management, patient safety, or anyone else.

Although responders were people to whom workers naturally gravitated for advice and support, and the programme was designed to be accessible and convenient, in the initial years after the programme launched it received very few calls. In retrospect, there were problems with implementation. After this initial launch, and lower than expected utilisation of the programme, a needs analysis was conducted to understand barriers that may exist to access and use of the RISE programme resources (Pillar 1). Three important barriers to using RISE were identified:

- lack of recognition of the high prevalence of the second victim phenomenon in hospital workers
- lack of knowledge that the programme exists and is intended for them
- the natural aversion of healthcare workers to ask for help, which many have internalised as showing weakness.

At a minimum, taking action to overcome these barriers would have required greater efforts in marketing and education, neither of which was delivered sufficiently in the early programme. In the initial phase of the RISE rollout, some efforts were made to engage staff. Members of the development team delivered presentations at staff meetings on nursing units in the hospital. The presentations featured some of the origin stories for patient safety at the Johns Hopkins Hospital, and how these critical incidents adversely affected providers. While these presentations engaged some of the staff, many more staff members were never reached. After the initial meetings, presentations were not repeated regularly, even on units with the highest patient acuity. Some units never received a formal presentation or other education. Insufficient attention to the engagement and education decreased the likelihood that individuals or their managers would activate RISE when it was needed – the actual execution of the intervention.

Evaluation posed an additional problem (Pillar 4).[122] Because of the potentially sensitive nature of patient adverse events, a top priority for the development team was to emphasise the confidentiality of the programme. The team thought that to use the programme, healthcare workers would need to feel that it was safe. Therefore, the programme did not collect identifying information on callers, and did not follow up systematically. Although this may have been necessary to reassure potential users, it made it impossible to collect representative data on user experience of the programme.

In subsequent years, these barriers received greater attention, and increased efforts were devoted to engaging and educating as many of the healthcare staff at the hospital as possible. RISE and the second victim phenomenon began to get broader attention from hospital leadership and media channels. Screensavers with information about RISE were added to every computer screen in the hospital, to reinforce messages delivered in training (Pillar 5). RISE played an important role following several high-profile adverse events and was recognised for this. The COVID-19 pandemic demonstrated the near-universal prevalence of distress among hospital staff members, and helped to normalise the use of RISE and other supporting resources.[121] Marketing and communications teams mounted a campaign to publicise the availability of services and how to reach them. All this led to much greater willingness to call RISE and receive support. Increased emotional engagement of health workers was accompanied by the incorporation of material related to staff wellbeing and support into the formal curriculum. These topics were introduced into the patient safety course taught to every second-year medical student, as well as to some nursing students.[123] They were also added to the orientation for new house officers in the major specialties. Optional training in psychological first aid was offered to interns and residents. This alignment of RISE training with existing training programmes was critical for achieving broad awareness.

In summary, RISE was an intervention designed to improve the well-being of healthcare workers, and indirectly the quality of care they deliver, patient safety, and outcomes.[124] The implementation of RISE would have benefitted from a more systematic application of the training needs analysis early in its development process. In this case, key elements include identification of barriers to successful implementation and efforts to overcome them.

5 Critiques of Training as an Improvement Approach

Education and training can be powerful tools for change and improvement but have limitations and weaknesses. Some are inherent in the methods (e.g. transfer of training from the learning environment to the work environment is always challenging), and some are related to misuse (e.g. failure to follow evidence-based practices for design and delivery) or abuse (e.g. use of training when it is not the right solution). Next, we explore recurring themes in inherent limitations, misuse, and abuse of education and training as an approach to healthcare improvement and provide thoughts on future directions of research and application to address these challenges and gaps.

5.1 Training Interventions Are Resource-Intensive

Well-developed training that adheres to the principles and practices outlined previously requires several key resources, all of which are scarce and costly. First, expertise in the training development process itself is required. Larger organisations may have skilled instructional designers, programme evaluators, and other educators, but smaller organisations often do not. Second, there is growing empirical literature indicating that the quality of the trainer impacts outcomes.[125] Skilled and effective trainers may be a rate-limiting factor in disseminating effective training. Third, and likely to be most important, the end users of training programmes (i.e. the frontline healthcare workforce) are experiencing increased workload, staff shortages, shifting role structures and a rapid pace of change (i.e. the 'shelf life' of knowledge and skills is decreasing), and a large volume of updates to evidence-based practices. These factors appear to create conditions where the need for education and training has never been greater, but the available time of staff to participate has never been a scarcer resource.

Future research in this area will involve technology-driven solutions to increase the efficiency of the design, delivery, and evaluation of training. Just-in-time training, particularly pre-procedure simulations, is one means to reduce overall time spent in dedicated training and to minimise the time between learning and performance. While evidence of effectiveness remains sparse, studies suggest this may be an effective and time-saving approach.[126] The often promised, yet infrequently documented, efficiency gains of artificial intelligence will no doubt occupy researchers for years to come. Applications relevant to training and education include automated training needs analysis (automating the analysis of relevant research, policies and procedure guides to define competencies, and learning objectives), and serving the role of tutors or coaches in personalised and interactive training programmes.[127–129] If proven effective, these approaches could dramatically reduce the burdens of developing and implementing training programmes.

5.2 Alignment across Training Programmes Is Challenging

Education and training programmes are often designed in relative isolation from one another and may fail to connect in important ways. As training programmes grow in number, they should (but frequently fail to) reinforce and elaborate upon one another – for example, when they target related competences. Some progress has been made in consolidating competency models across professions and geography, but much remains to be done. This lack of alignment compounds the challenges of resource scarcity described earlier, as much of the work of training design is replicated across different training programmes instead of pulling from or linking to existing and related resources (e.g. needs analyses or competency models created for different, but very related training efforts).

In addition to continued maturation of quality and safety as concepts in health profession education, future research to address this challenge will have to involve individual organisations creating more sophisticated and integrated strategic approaches to learning, including both formal training and informal learning strategies.[130] The solutions to the challenge of alignment involve organisations providing a consolidated and integrated approach to learning and development that informs the design and delivery of each individual learning experience or training event.

5.3 Training Is a Misused and Abused Method

In healthcare improvement, one of the most often violated of the 13 principles introduced in this Element is Principle 2: Confirm that training is the best solution. Despite being resource-intensive, training is often a default response to operational challenges or risks, even when other solutions (e.g. work process, technology, or policy changes) would be more effective. Many times, low-quality training is offered as a poorly conceived solution to a multifaceted problem. Training is, for example, one of the most common recommendations resulting from root cause analysis,[131] and often is an action taken for the sake of action, especially as low-quality training that skips many if not all evidence-based design practices can be created and fielded quickly. This has led to the characterisation of training as a low-value improvement method,[132] but higher-quality training programmes, used more judiciously and focused on clear knowledge, skill, or attitude gaps, would likely have a larger effect.

Future research to address this challenge requires developing more practical methods of task and needs analysis. Many of the traditional methods (e.g. hierarchical task analysis) are time-intensive and may not yield insight into the broader system, where other interventions could more effectively improve overall system performance. Human factors researchers have noted these limitations of current approaches, and research on more effective approaches is ongoing.[133] Additionally, developing reporting standards for training interventions in quality or safety improvement studies will enable synthesis of evidence that could inform more general guidance on the tasks or conditions under which training is most likely to be an effective intervention.

6 Conclusions

Healthcare delivery systems rely on the expertise of dedicated professionals. Formal education and training are central methods for building and maintaining that expertise, and are one of the primary mechanisms that organisations use to cultivate their performance and improvement capacities. Existing literature provides good guidance for how to design, deliver, and evaluate effective training. However, pressures in the workplace are creating the need to rethink how to practically deliver effective learning interventions. But the needs are clear. For developing healthcare improvement professionals and leaders, education programmes are and will remain critical for building the complex set of technical and adaptive capabilities needed to affect change in healthcare settings. For specific healthcare improvement projects, training is often one component of a broader change intervention. Adhering to the evidence-based principles outlined here can help ensure the overall success of the programme.

7 Further Reading

- Salas et al.[27] provide more specific details on the content in Section 3 of this Element.
- Thomas et al.[10] provide a practical approach to developing curricula for medical education that is broadly applicable to foundational educational activities.
- Kraiger and Ford[17] provide a comprehensive review of training studies, and discuss future direction for research as well as offering a synthesis of the science helpful for guiding the development of a strategic learning plan for an organisation.
- The Canadian Patient Safety Institute[84] report is an example of efforts to integrate patient safety competencies across the health professions.
- Kraiger and colleagues[9] provide well-researched broad guidance and a valuable resource on many issues in training and development in organisations.

Soong and Shojania[132] discuss many of the common misuses and abuses of training as a healthcare improvement method, offering a helpful reminder of what not to do with training and emphasising that training is one of the many tools for improving quality and safety.

Contributors

LEB, AWW, and MAR contributed to initial outlines, drafting, and editing of the manuscript. AWW and MAR have approved the final version.

Conflicts of Interest

None.

Acknowledgements

We thank the peer reviewers for their insightful comments and recommendations to improve the Element. A list of peer reviewers is published at www.cambridge.org/IQ-peer-reviewers.

Funding

This Element was funded by THIS Institute (The Healthcare Improvement Studies Institute, www.thisinstitute.cam.ac.uk). THIS Institute is strengthening the evidence base for improving the quality and safety of healthcare. THIS Institute is supported by a grant to the University of Cambridge from the Health Foundation – an independent charity committed to bringing about better health and healthcare for people in the United Kingdom.

About the Authors

Lauren E. Benishek was an organisational psychologist and patient safety researcher who focused on the power of relationships to improve wellness and safety. She passed away prior to the final publication of this manuscript and is missed greatly by her colleagues.

Albert W. Wu is a health services researcher studying the impact of safety problems on patients and health care workers, and on patient reported outcomes. He is Director of the Center for Health Services and Outcomes Research (CHSOR), and Editor in Chief of Journal of Patient Safety and Risk Management.

Michael A. Rosen is a human factors psychologist studying how teams and technology enable safe operations. Simulation for both analysis and improvement is central to his work. He is Director of Research at the Armstrong Institute for Patient Safety and Quality, and the Johns Hopkins School of Medicine Simulation Centre.

Creative Commons License

The online version of this work is published under a Creative Commons licence called CC-BY-NC-ND 4.0 (https://creativecommons.org/licenses/by-nc-nd/4.0). It means that you're free to reuse this work. In fact, we encourage it. We just ask that you acknowledge THIS Institute as the creator, you don't distribute a modified version without our permission, and you don't sell it or use it for any activity that generates revenue without our permission. Ultimately, we want our work to have impact. So if you've got a use in mind but you're not sure it's allowed, just ask us at enquiries@thisinstitute.cam.ac.uk.

The printed version is subject to statutory exceptions and to the provisions of relevant licensing agreements, so you will need written permission from Cambridge University Press to reproduce any part of it.

All versions of this work may contain content reproduced under licence from third parties. You must obtain permission to reproduce this content from these third parties directly.

References

1. Barsuk JH, Cohen ER, Feinglass J, McGaghie WC, Wayne DB. Use of simulation-based education to reduce catheter-related bloodstream infections. *Arch Intern Med* 2009; 169(15): 1420–3. https://doi.org/10.1001/archinternmed.2009.215.
2. Schmutz JB, Meier LL, Manser T. How effective is teamwork really? The relationship between teamwork and performance in healthcare teams: A systematic review and meta-analysis. *BMJ Open* 2019; 9(9): e028280. https://doi.org/10.1136/bmjopen-2018-028280.
3. Halligan M, Zecevic A. Safety culture in healthcare: A review of concepts, dimensions, measures and progress. *BMJ Qual Saf* 2011; 20(4): 338–43. https://doi.org/10.1136/bmjqs.2010.040964.
4. McFadden KL, Stock GN, Gowen CR, 3rd. Leadership, safety climate, and continuous quality improvement: Impact on process quality and patient safety. *Health Care Manage Rev* 2015; 40(1): 24–34. https://doi.org/10.1097/HMR.0000000000000006.
5. Cooke M, Ironside PM, Ogrinc GS. Mainstreaming quality and safety: A reformulation of quality and safety education for health professions students. *BMJ Qual Saf* 2011; 20 Suppl 1(Suppl_1): i79–82. https://doi.org/10.1136/bmjqs.2010.046516.
6. McGaghie WC, Hinkamp MM, Harden RM. *International Best Practices for Evaluation in the Health Professions*. London: Radcliffe; 2022. https://doi.org/10.1201/9781846198557.
7. Ritter FE, Nerb J, Lehtinen E, O'Shea T. *In Order to Learn*. Oxford: Oxford University Press; 2007. https://doi.org/10.1093/acprof:oso/9780195178845.001.0001
8. Nestel D, Kelly M, Jolly B, Watson M. *Healthcare Simulation Education*. Oxford: John Wiley & Sons; 2017. https://doi.org/10.1002/9781119061656.
9. Kraiger K, Passmore J, Santos NRd, Malvezzi S. *The Wiley Blackwell Handbook of the Psychology of Training, Development, and Performance Improvement*. Oxford: John Wiley & Sons; 2014. https://doi.org/10.1002/9781118736982.
10. Thomas PA, Kern DE, Hughes MT, Chen BY. *Curriculum Development for Medical Education: A Six-Step Approach*. Baltimore, MA: JHU Press; 2016.

11. Bell BS, Tannenbaum SI, Ford JK, Noe RA, Kraiger K. 100 years of training and development research: What we know and where we should go. *J Appl Psychol* 2017; 102(3): 305–23. https://doi.org/10.1037/apl0000142.
12. Campbell JP. Personnel Training and Development. *Annu Rev Psychol* 1971; 22(1): 565–602. https://doi.org/10.1146/annurev.ps.22.020171.003025.
13. Salas E, Cannon-Bowers JA. The science of training: A decade of progress. *Annu Rev Psychol* 2001; 52(1): 471–99. https://doi.org/10.1146/annurev.psych.52.1.471.
14. Salas E, Tannenbaum SI, Kraiger K, Smith-Jentsch KA. The science of training and development in organizations: What matters in practice. *Psychol Sci Public Interest* 2012; 13(2): 74–101. https://doi.org/10.1177/1529100612436661
15. Ford JK, Baldwin TT, Prasad J. Transfer of training: The known and the unknown. *Annu Rev Organ Psychol Organ Behav* 2018; 5(1): 201–25. https://doi.org/10.1146/annurev-orgpsych-032117-104443.
16. Goldstein, IL, Ford JK. *Training in Organizations: Needs Assessment, Development, and Evaluation*, 4th ed. Belmont, CA: Wadsworth; 2002.
17. Kraiger K, Ford JK. The science of workplace instruction: Learning and development applied to work. *Annu Rev Organ Psychol Organ Behav* 2021; 8(1): 45–72. https://doi.org/10.1146/annurev-orgpsych-012420-060109.
18. Salas E, Stagl KC. Design training systematically and follow the science of training. In EA Locke, (ed.), *Handbook of Principles of Organizational Behavior: Indispensible Knowledge for Evidence-Based Management*. Oxford: John Wiley & Sons; 2009: 59–84. https://doi.org/10.1002/9781119206422.ch4.
19. Alliger GM, Tannenbaum SI, Bennett W, Traver H, Shotland A. A meta-analysis of the relations among training criteria. *Pers Psychol* 2006; 50(2): 341–58. https://doi.org/10.1111/j.1744-6570.1997.tb00911.x.
20. Sitzmann T, Brown KG, Casper WJ, Ely K, Zimmerman RD. A review and meta-analysis of the nomological network of trainee reactions. *J Appl Psychol*. 2008; 93(2): 280–95. https://doi.org/10.1037/0021-9010.93.2.280.
21. Garavan T, McCarthy A, Sheehan M et al. Measuring the organizational impact of training: The need for greater methodological rigor. *Hum Resour Dev Q* 2019; 30(3): 291–309. https://doi.org/10.1002/hrdq.21345.
22. Hughes AM, Gregory ME, Joseph DL et al. Saving lives: A meta-analysis of team training in healthcare. *J Appl Psychol*. 2016; 101(9): 1266–304. https://doi.org/10.1037/apl0000120.
23. Murad MH, Coto-Yglesias F, Varkey P, Prokop LJ, Murad AL. The effectiveness of self-directed learning in health professions education: a

systematic review. *Med Educ* 2010; 44(11): 1057–68. https://doi.org/10.1111/j.1365-2923.2010.03750.x.
24. Aslaksen K, Lorås H. Matching instruction with modality-specific learning style: Effects on immediate recall and working memory performance. *Edu Sciences* 2019; 9(1): 32. https://doi.org/ARTN3210.3390/educsci9010032.
25. Aslaksen K, Loras H. The modality-specific learning style hypothesis: A mini-review. *Front Psychol* 2018; 9: 1538. https://doi.org/10.3389/fpsyg.2018.01538.
26. Baldwin T, Magjuka RJ. Organizational context and training effectiveness: Improving training effectiveness in work organizations. *Psychol Press*; 2014; 111–40. https://doi.org/10.4324/9781315806662.
27. Salas E. *Team Training Essentials*. Oxford: Routledge; 2015. https://doi.org/10.4324/9781315747644.
28. Wong BM, Etchells EE, Kuper A, Levinson W, Shojania KG. Teaching quality improvement and patient safety to trainees: A systematic review. *Acad Med* 2010; 85(9): 1425–39. https://doi.org/10.1097/ACM.0b013e3181e2d0c6.
29. Campion MA, Fink AA, Ruggeberg BJ et al. Doing competencies well: Best practices in competency modeling. *Pers Psychol* 2011; 64(1): 225–62. https://doi.org/10.1111/j.1744-6570.2010.01207.x.
30. Moran KM, Harris IB, Valenta AL. Competencies for patient safety and quality improvement: A synthesis of recommendations in influential position papers. *Jt Comm J Qual Patient Saf* 2016; 42(4): 162–9. https://doi.org/10.1016/s1553-7250(16)42020-9.
31. Langins M, Borgermans L. Strengthening a competent health workforce for the provision of coordinated/integrated health services. *Int J Integrated Care* 2016; 16(6): A321. https://doi.org/10.5334/ijic.2779.
32. Tregunno D, Ginsburg L, Clarke B, Norton P. Integrating patient safety into health professionals' curricula: A qualitative study of medical, nursing and pharmacy faculty perspectives. *BMJ Qual Saf* 2014; 23(3): 257–64. https://doi.org/10.1136/bmjqs-2013-001900.
33. Albarqouni L, Hoffmann T, Straus S et al. Core competencies in evidence-based practice for health professionals: Consensus statement based on a systematic review and delphi survey. *JAMA Netw Open* 2018; 1(2): e180281. https://doi.org/10.1001/jamanetworkopen.2018.0281.
34. Olson A, Rencic J, Cosby K et al. Competencies for improving diagnosis: An interprofessional framework for education and training in health care. *Diagnosis* 2019; 6(4): 335–41. https://doi.org/10.1515/dx-2018-0107.
35. Mathura P, Lee DH, Thompson A, McMurtry N, Kassam N. Providing quality improvement training in an advanced pharmacy practice experience

elective. *Curr Pharm Teach Learn* 2021; 13(4): 397–402. https://doi.org/10.1016/j.cptl.2020.11.013.

36. Brown A, Lafreniere K, Freedman D et al. A realist synthesis of quality improvement curricula in undergraduate and postgraduate medical education: What works, for whom, and in what contexts? *BMJ Qual Saf* 2021; 30(4): 337–52. https://doi.org/10.1136/bmjqs-2020-010887.

37. Wong BM, Baum KD, Headrick LA et al. Building the bridge to quality: An urgent call to integrate quality improvement and patient safety education with clinical care. *Acad Med* 2020; 95(1): 59–68. https://doi.org/10.1097/ACM.0000000000002937.

38. Durstenfeld MS, Statman S, Carney K et al. Swimming with sharks: Teaching residents value-based medicine and quality improvement through resident-pitched projects. *J Grad Med Educ* 2020; 12(3): 320–6. https://doi.org/10.4300/JGME-D-19-00421.1.

39. Wahlberg KJ, Burnett M, Muthukrishnan P et al. Partnering with patients in a quality improvement curriculum for internal medicine residents. *J Patient Exp* 2021; 8: 2374373521999604. https://doi.org/10.1177/2374373521999604.

40. Chen A, Wolpaw BJ, Vande Vusse LK et al. Creating a framework to integrate residency program and medical center approaches to quality improvement and patient safety training. *Acad Med* 2021; 96(1): 75–82. https://doi.org/10.1097/ACM.0000000000003725.

41. Rosen MA, Salas E, Pavlas D et al. Demonstration-based training: A review of instructional features. *Hum Factors* 2010; 52(5): 596–609. https://doi.org/10.1177/0018720810381071.

42. Brazil V, Purdy E, Bajaj K. *Simulation as an Improvement Technique*. Cambridge: Cambridge University Press; 2023. www.cambridge.org/core/product/27E6D4C656EAB32476EE582186072551.

43. Goodwin CDG, Velasquez E, Ross J et al. Development of a novel and scalable simulation-based teamwork training model using within-group debriefing of observed video simulation. *Jt Comm J Qual Patient Saf* 2021; 47(6): 385–91. https://doi.org/10.1016/j.jcjq.2021.02.006.

44. Branzetti JB, Adedipe AA, Gittinger MJ et al. Randomised controlled trial to assess the effect of a Just-in-Time training on procedural performance: A proof-of-concept study to address procedural skill decay. *BMJ Qual Saf* 2017; 26(11): 881–91. https://doi.org/10.1136/bmjqs-2017-006656.

45. Nishisaki A, Donoghue AJ, Colborn S et al. Effect of just-in-time simulation training on tracheal intubation procedure safety in the pediatric intensive care unit. *Anesthesiology* 2010; 113(1): 214–23. https://doi.org/10.1097/ALN.0b013e3181e19bf2.

46. Clarke B, Haze N, Sly J et al. Just-in-time safety training for N95 respirators: A virtual approach. *Nurs Manage* 2020; 51(11): 17–22. https://doi.org/10.1097/01.NUMA.0000719392.56384.46.
47. Thompson L, Lin F, Faithfull-Byrne A, et al. Clinical coaches and patient safety – Just in time: A descriptive exploratory study. *Nurse Educ Pract* 2021; 54: 103–34. https://doi.org/10.1016/j.nepr.2021.103134.
48. Pronovost PJ, Marsteller JA. Creating a fractal-based quality management infrastructure. *J Health Organ Manag* 2014; 28(4): 576–86. https://doi.org/10.1108/jhom-11-2013-0262.
49. O'Leary KJ, Afsar-Manesh N, Budnitz T, Dunn AS, Myers JS. Hospital quality and patient safety competencies: Development, description, and recommendations for use. *J Hosp Med* 2011; 6(9): 530–6. https://doi.org/10.1002/jhm.937.
50. Vana PK, Vottero BA, Christie-McAuliffe CA. *Introduction to Quality and Safety Education for Nurses: Core Competencies for Nursing Leadership and Management*. New York City: Springer; 2018.
51. Myers JS, Lane-Fall MB, Perfetti RH, et al. Demonstrating the value of postgraduate fellowships for physicians in quality improvement and patient safety. *BMJ Qual Saf.* 2020; 29(8): 645–54. https://doi.org/10.1136/bmjqs-2019-010204.
52. Heifetz RA, Laurie DL. The work of leadership. *Harv Bus Rev* 1997; 75(1): 124–34.
53. Kotter JP. What leaders really do. *Harv Bus Rev* 2001; 79(11): 85–95.
54. Goldman J, Wong BM. Nothing soft about 'soft skills': Core competencies in quality improvement and patient safety education and practice. *BMJ Qual Saf* 2020; 29(8): 619–22. https://doi.org/10.1136/bmjqs-2019-010512.
55. Kelly S, Redmond P, King S et al. Training in the use of intrapartum electronic fetal monitoring with cardiotocography: Systematic review and meta-analysis. *BJOG: Int J Obstet Gynaecol* 2021; 128(9): 1408–19.
56. Amaral C, Sequeira C, Albacar-Riobóo N et al. Patient safety training programs for health care professionals: A scoping review. *J Patient Saf* 2023; 19(1): 48–58.
57. Gregory M, Feitosa J, Driskell T, Salas E, Vessey W. Designing, delivering, and evaluating team training in organizations: Principles that work. Developing and enhancing teamwork in organizations: evidence-based practice guidelines edn. Edited by Salas E, Tannenbum S, Cohen D, Latham G San Francisco, CA: Wiley. 2013.
58. Gould D, Kelly D, White I, Chidgey J. Training needs analysis: A literature review and reappraisal. *Int J Nurs Stud* 2004; 41(5): 471–86. https://doi.org/10.1016/j.ijnurstu.2003.12.003.

59. Moore ML, Dutton P. Training needs analysis: Review and critique. *Acad Manage Rev* 1978; 3(3): 532–45.
60. Taylor PJ, O'Driscoll MP. A new integrated framework for training needs analysis. *Hum Resour Manag J* 1998; 8(2): 29.
61. Sleezer CM, Russ-Eft DF, Gupta K. *A Practical Guide to Needs Assessment, 3rd ed.* San Francisco, CA: Wiley; 2014. https://doi.org/10.1002/9781118826164.
62. Brannick MT, Levine EL, Morgeson FP. *Job and Work Analysis: Methods, Research, and Applications for Human Resource Management.* London: Sage; 2007.
63. Manuele FA. Achieving risk reduction, effectively. *PSEP* 2006; 84(B3): 184–90. https://doi.org/10.1205/psep.05083.
64. Health NIfOSa. Hierarchy of Controls 2015. www.cdc.gov/niosh/topics/hierarchy/default.html.
65. Practices IfSM. Medication Error Prevention 'Toolbox' 1999. www.ismp.org/resources/medication-error-prevention-toolbox.
66. Nishiyama C, Iwami T, Murakami Y et al. Effectiveness of simplified 15-min refresher BLS training program: A randomized controlled trial. *Resuscitation* 2015; 90: 56–60. https://doi.org/10.1016/j.resuscitation.2015.02.015.
67. Liberati EG, Peerally MF, Dixon-Woods M. Learning from high risk industries may not be straightforward: A qualitative study of the hierarchy of risk controls approach in healthcare. *Int J Qual Health Care* 2018; 30(1): 39–43.
68. Lotfinejad N, Peters A, Tartari E et al. Hand hygiene in health care: 20 years of ongoing advances and perspectives. *Lancet Infect Dis* 2021; 21(8): e209–e21. https://doi.org/10.1016/S1473-3099(21)00383-2.
69. Stanton NA. Hierarchical task analysis: Developments, applications, and extensions. *Appl Ergon* 2006; 37(1): 55–79. https://doi.org/10.1016/j.apergo.2005.06.003.
70. Schuler D, Namioka A. *Participatory Design: Principles and Practices.* London: CRC Press; 1993.
71. Blume BD, Ford JK, Baldwin TT, Huang JL. Transfer of training: A meta-analytic review. *J Manage* 2010; 36(4): 1065–105. https://doi.org/10.1177/0149206309352880.
72. Lyubovnikova J, West THR, Dawson JF, West MA. Examining the indirect effects of perceived organizational support for teamwork training on acute health care team productivity and innovation: The role of shared objectives. *Group Organ Manage* 2018; 43(3): 382–413. https://doi.org/10.1177/1059601118769742.

73. Pronovost PJ, Berenholtz SM, Needham DM. Translating evidence into practice: A model for large scale knowledge translation. *BMJ* 2008; 337- (7676): a1714. https://doi.org/10.1136/bmj.a1714.
74. Pitts SI, Maruthur NM, Luu NP et al. Implementing the comprehensive unit-based safety program (CUSP) to improve patient safety in an academic primary care practice. *Jt Comm J Qual Patient Saf* 2017; 43(11): 591–7. https://doi.org/10.1016/j.jcjq.2017.06.006.
75. Noe R, Colquitt J. Planning for training impact: Principles of training effectiveness. In K Kraiger (ed.), *Creating Implementing, and Maintaining Effective Training and Development: State-of-the-art Lesson for Practice*. San Francisco, CA: Jossey-Bass; 2002: 77–84.
76. Sitzmann T, Bell BS, Kraiger K, Kanar AM. A multilevel analysis of the effect of prompting self-regulation in technology-delivered instruction. *Pers Psychol* 2009; 62(4): 697–734. https://doi.org/10.1111/j.1744-6570.2009.01155.x.
77. Awais Bhatti M, Kaur S. The role of individual and training design factors on training transfer. *J Eur Ind Train* 2010; 34(7): 656–72.
78. Bandura A. *Self-efficacy: The Exercise of Control*. New York: W.H. Freeman; 1997.
79. Bloom B. *Taxonomy of Educational Objectives: The Classification of Educational Goals*. New York: Longmans, Green; 1956.
80. Krathwohl DR. A revision of bloom's taxonomy: An overview. *Theory Pract* 2010; 41(4): 212–8. https://doi.org/10.1207/s15430421tip4104_2.
81. Chatterjee D, Corral J. How to write well-defined learning objectives. *J Educ Perioper Med* 2017; 19(4): E610.
82. Knebel E, Greiner AC. *Health Professions Education: A Bridge to Quality*. Washington, DC: National Academies Press (US); 2003. https://doi.org/10.17226/10681.
83. America CoQoHCi. *Crossing the Quality Chasm: A New Health System for the 21st Century*. Washington, DC: National Academies Press; 2001.
84. Canadian Patient Safety Institute. *The Safety Competencies: Enhancing Patient Safety Across the Health Professions*. Edmonton, Alberta: Canadian Patient Safety Institute; 2020.
85. Bandura A. *Social Learning Theory*. Oxford, England: Prentic-Hall; 1977.
86. D'Angelo A-L, Kchir H. *Error Management Training in Medical Simulation*. Treasure Island, FL: StatPearls Publishing; 2019.
87. Keith N, Frese M. Effectiveness of error management training: A meta-analysis. *J Appl Psychol* 2008; 93(1): 59–69. https://doi.org/10.1037/0021-9010.93.1.59.

88. Metcalfe J. Learning from errors. *Annu Rev Psychol* 2017; 68: 465–89. https://doi.org/10.1146/annurev-psych-010416-044022.
89. Kirkpatrick D. Evaluation. In C RL (ed.), *Training and Development Handbook*. 2nd ed. New York: McGraw Hill; 1976: 294–312.
90. Kirkpatrick D. *Evaluating Training Programs: The Four Levels*. San Francisco, CA: Berrett-Kichler; 1994.
91. Phillips JJ. *Return on Investment*. Houston, TX: Gulf; 1997.
92. Phillips JJ, Phillips PP. *Handbook of Training Evaluation and Measurement Methods*: Oxford: Routledge; 2016.
93. Phillips PP, Phillips JJ. Return on investment. In KH Silber, WR Foshay, R Watkins et al. (eds.), *Handbook of Improving Performance in the Workplace: Volumes 1-3*. Oxford: Wiley; 2009: 823–46. https://doi.org/10.1002/9780470592663.ch53.
94. Patterson F, Zibarras L and Ashworth V. Situational judgement tests in medical education and training: Research, theory and practice: AMEE Guide No. 100. *Med Teach* 2016; 38(1): 3–17. https://doi.org/10.3109/0142159X.2015.1072619.
95. Okuyama A, Martowirono K, Bijnen B. Assessing the patient safety competencies of healthcare professionals: A systematic review. *BMJ Qual Saf* 2011; 20(11): 991–1000. https://doi.org/10.1136/bmjqs-2011-000148.
96. Smith-Jentsch KA, Salas E, Brannick MT. To transfer or not to transfer? Investigating the combined effects of trainee characteristics, team leader support, and team climate. *J Appl Psychol* 2001; 86(2): 279–92. https://doi.org/10.1037/0021-9010.86.2.279.
97. Morgenroth T, Ryan MK, Peters K. The motivational theory of role modeling: How role models influence role aspirants' goals. *Rev Gen Psychol* 2015; 19(4): 465–83. https://doi.org/10.1037/gpr0000059.
98. Clarke N. Job/work environment factors influencing training transfer within a human service agency: Some indicative support for Baldwin and Ford's transfer climate construct. *Int J Train Dev* 2002; 6(3): 146–62. https://doi.org/10.1111/1468-2419.00156.
99. Burke LA, Hutchins HM. Training transfer: An integrative literature review. *Hum Res Dev Rev* 2007; 6(3): 263–96. https://doi.org/10.1177/1534484307303035.
100. Lazzara EH, Benishek LE, Hughes AM et al. Enhancing the organization's workforce: Guidance for effective training sustainment. *Consult Psych J* 2021; 73(1): 1–26. https://doi.org/10.1037/cpb0000185.
101. Lee J, Lee H, Kim S et al. Debriefing methods and learning outcomes in simulation nursing education: A systematic review and meta-analysis.

Nurse Educ Today 2020; 87: 104345. https://doi.org/10.1016/j.nedt.2020.104345.

102. Rai A, Ghosh P, Chauhan R, Singh R. Improving in-role and extra-role performances with rewards and recognition: Does engagement mediate the process? *Manag Res Rev* 2018; 41(8): 902–19. https://doi.org/10.1108/Mrr-12-2016-0280.

103. Ford JK, Wroten SP. Introducing new methods for conducting training evaluation and for linking training evaluation to program redesign. *Pers Psychol* 1984; 37(4): 651–65. https://doi.org/10.1111/j.1744-6570.1984.tb00531.x.

104. Draycott T, Sibanda T, Owen L et al. Does training in obstetric emergencies improve neonatal outcome? *BJOG: Int J Obstet Gynaecol* 2006; 113(2): 177–82.

105. Foundation P. PROMPT's Story 2024. www.promptmaternity.org/prompt-uk-1.

106. Siassakos D, Fox R, Crofts JF et al. The management of a simulated emergency: Better teamwork, better performance. *Resuscitation* 2011; 82(2): 203–6. https://doi.org/10.1016/j.resuscitation.2010.10.029.

107. Weiner CP. Reassuringly expensive – A commentary on obstetric emergency training in high-resource settings. *Best Pract Res Clin Obstet Gynaecol* 2022; 80: 14–24. https://doi.org/10.1016/j.bpobgyn.2021.11.009.

108. Salas E, Rosen MA, King H. Managing teams managing crises: Principles of teamwork to improve patient safety in the Emergency Room and beyond. *Theor Issues Ergon Sci* 2007; 8(5): 381–94 https://doi.org/10.1080/14639220701317764.

109. Winter C, Crofts J, Draycott T, Muchatuta N. *PROMPT Course Manual*. Cambridge: Cambridge University Press; 2017

110. Shoushtarian M, Barnett M, McMahon F, Ferris J. Impact of introducing practical obstetric multi-professional training (PROMPT) into maternity units in victoria, Australia. *BJOG: Int J Obstet Gynaecol* 2014; 121(13): 1710–8.

111. Ghag K, Bahl R, Winter C et al. Key components influencing the sustainability of a multi-professional obstetric emergencies training programme in a middle-income setting: A qualitative study. *BMC Health Serv Res* 2021; 21(1): 384 https://doi.org/10.1186/s12913-021-06385-5.

112. Brogaard L, Glerup Lauridsen K, Lofgren B et al. The effects of obstetric emergency team training on patient outcome: A systematic review and meta-analysis. *Acta Obstet Gynecol Scand* 2022; 101(1): 25–36. https://doi.org/10.1111/aogs.14263.

113. Hunt EA, Jeffers J, McNamara L et al. Improved Cardiopulmonary Resuscitation Performance With CODE ACES(2): A Resuscitation Quality Bundle. *J Am Heart Assoc* 2018; 7(24): e009860. https://doi.org/10.1161/JAHA.118.009860.
114. Keiser NL, Arthur W. A meta-analysis of the effectiveness of the after-action review (or debrief) and factors that influence its effectiveness. *J Appl Psychol* 2021; 106(7): 1007–32. https://doi.org/10.1037/apl0000821.
115. Kolbe M, Eppich W, Rudolph J et al. Managing psychological safety in debriefings: A dynamic balancing act. *BMJ Simul Technol Enhanc Learn* 2020; 6(3): 164–71. https://doi.org/10.1136/bmjstel-2019-000470
116. Hunt EA, Cruz-Eng H, Bradshaw JH et al. A novel approach to life support training using 'action-linked phrases'. *Resuscitation* 2015; 86: 1–5.
117. Sullivan NJ, Duval-Arnould JM, Perretta JS, Rosen MA, Hunt EA. Using simulation to design choreography for a cardiopulmonary arrest response. *Clin Simul Nurs* 2015; 11(11): 489–93 https://doi.org/10.1016/j.ecns.2015.10.004.
118. Wu AW. Medical error: The second victim. *BMJ* 2000; 18; 320(7237): 726–7. https://doi.org/10.1136/bmj.320.7237.726.
119. Busch IM, Scott SD, Connors C et al. The role of institution-based peer support for health care workers emotionally affected by workplace violence. *Jt Comm J Qual Patient Saf* 2021; 47(3): 146–56. https://doi.org/10.1016/j.jcjq.2020.11.005.
120. Edrees H, Connors C, Paine L et al. Implementing the RISE second victim support programme at the Johns Hopkins Hospital: A case study. *BMJ Open* 2016; 6(9): e011708. https://doi.org/10.1136/bmjopen-2016-011708.
121. Wu AW, Buckle P, Haut ER et al. Supporting the emotional well-being of health care workers during the COVID-19 pandemic. *J Patient Saf Risk Manag* 2020; 25(3): 93–6 https://doi.org/10.1177/2516043520931971.
122. Connors CA, Dukhanin V, Norvell M, Wu AW. RISE: Exploring volunteer retention and sustainability of a second victim support program. *J Healthc Manag* 2021; 66(1): 19–32 https://doi.org/10.1097/JHM-D-19-00264.
123. Aboumatar HJ, Thompson D, Wu A et al. Development and evaluation of a 3-day patient safety curriculum to advance knowledge, self-efficacy and system thinking among medical students. *BMJ Qual Saf* 2012; 21(5): 416–22. https://doi.org/10.1136/bmjqs-2011-000463.
124. Wu AW. My eye – The importance of clinician well-being in 2020. *J Patient Saf Risk Manag* 2020; 25(1): 3–4. https://doi.org/10.1177/2516043520903513.

125. Glerum DR, Joseph DL, McKenny AF, Fritzsche BA. The trainer matters: Cross-classified models of trainee reactions. *J Appl Psychol* 2021; 106(2): 281–99. https://doi.org/10.1037/apl0000503
126. Patocka C, Pandya A, Brennan E et al. The impact of just-in-time simulation training for healthcare professionals on learning and performance outcomes: A systematic review. *Simul Healthc* 2024; 19(1S): S32–S40. https://doi.org/10.1097/SIH.0000000000000764.
127. Bhatt P, Muduli A. Artificial intelligence in learning and development: A systematic literature review. *Eur J Train and Devel* 2023; 47(7/8): 677–94. https://doi.org/10.1108/EJTD-09-2021-0143.
128. Chen Z. Artificial intelligence-virtual trainer: Innovative didactics aimed at personalized training needs. *J Knowl Econ* 2023; 14(2): 2007–25.
129. Maity S. Identifying opportunities for artificial intelligence in the evolution of training and development practices. *J Manag Devel* 2019; 38(8): 651–63. https://doi.org/10.1108/Jmd-03-2019-0069.
130. Aboumatar HJ, Weaver SJ, Rees D et al. Towards high-reliability organising in healthcare: A strategy for building organisational capacity. *BMJ Qual Saf* 2017; 26(8): 663–70. https://doi.org/10.1136/bmjqs-2016-006240.
131. Hibbert PD, Thomas MJW, Deakin A et al. Are root cause analyses recommendations effective and sustainable? An observational study. *Int J Qual Health Care* 2018; 30(2): 124–31. https://doi.org/10.1093/intqhc/mzx181.
132. Soong C, Shojania KG. Education as a low-value improvement intervention: Often necessary but rarely sufficient. *BMJ Qual Saf* 2020; 29(5): 353–357.
133. Holman M, Walker G, Lansdown T et al. The binary-based model (BBM) for improved human factors method selection. *Hum Factors* 2021; 63(8): 1408–36. https://doi.org/10.1177/0018720820926875.

Cambridge Elements

Improving Quality and Safety in Healthcare

Editors-in-Chief
Mary Dixon-Woods
THIS Institute (The Healthcare Improvement Studies Institute)

Mary is Director of THIS Institute and is the Health Foundation Professor of Healthcare Improvement Studies in the Department of Public Health and Primary Care at the University of Cambridge. Mary leads a programme of research focused on healthcare improvement, healthcare ethics, and methodological innovation in studying healthcare.

Graham Martin
THIS Institute (The Healthcare Improvement Studies Institute)

Graham is Director of Research at THIS Institute, leading applied research programmes and contributing to the institute's strategy and development. His research interests are in the organisation and delivery of healthcare, and particularly the role of professionals, managers, and patients and the public in efforts at organisational change.

Executive Editor
Katrina Brown
THIS Institute (The Healthcare Improvement Studies Institute)

Katrina was Communications Manager at THIS Institute, providing editorial expertise to maximise the impact of THIS Institute's research findings. She managed the project to produce the series until 2023.

Editorial Team
Sonja Marjanovic
RAND Europe

Sonja is Director of RAND Europe's healthcare innovation, industry, and policy research. Her work provides decision-makers with evidence and insights to support innovation and improvement in healthcare systems, and to support the translation of innovation into societal benefits for healthcare services and population health.

Tom Ling
RAND Europe

Tom is Head of Evaluation at RAND Europe and President of the European Evaluation Society, leading evaluations and applied research focused on the key challenges facing health services. His current health portfolio includes evaluations of the innovation landscape, quality improvement, communities of practice, patient flow, and service transformation.

Ellen Perry
THIS Institute (The Healthcare Improvement Studies Institute)

Ellen supported the production of the series during 2020–21.

Gemma Petley
THIS Institute (The Healthcare Improvement Studies Institute)

Gemma is Senior Communications and Editorial Manager at THIS Institute, responsible for overseeing the production and maximising the impact of the series.

Claire Dipple
THIS Institute (The Healthcare Improvement Studies Institute)

Claire is Editorial Project Manager at THIS Institute, responsible for editing and projectmanaging the series.

About the Series

The past decade has seen enormous growth in both activity and research on improvement in healthcare. This series offers a comprehensive and authoritative set of overviews of the different improvement approaches available, exploring the thinking behind them, examining evidence for each approach, and identifying areas of debate.

Cambridge Elements

Improving Quality and Safety in Healthcare

Elements in the Series

Workplace Conditions
Jill Maben, Jane Ball, and Amy C. Edmondson

Governance and Leadership
Naomi J. Fulop and Angus I. G. Ramsay

Health Economics
Andrew Street and Nils Gutacker

Approaches to Spread, Scale-Up, and Sustainability
Chrysanthi Papoutsi, Trisha Greenhalgh, and Sonja Marjanovic

Statistical Process Control
Mohammed Amin Mohammed

Values and Ethics
Alan Cribb, Vikki Entwistle, and Polly Mitchell

Design Creativity
Gyuchan Thomas Jun, Sue Hignett and P. John Clarkson

Supply Chain Management
Sharon J. Williams

Measurement for Improvement
Alene Toulany and Kaveh G. Shojania

Learning Health Systems
Thomas Foley and Leora I. Horwitz

Clinical Microsystems and Team Coaching
Steve Harrison, Rachael Finn and Marjorie M. Godfrey

Audit, Feedback, and Behaviour Change
Noah Ivers and Robbie Foy

Education and Training as Improvement Interventions
Lauren E. Benishek, Albert W. Wu and Michael A. Rosen

A full series listing is available at: www.cambridge.org/IQ

Printed by Integrated Books International,
United States of America